Consumer Notes

Food Journal
And Diary

It's all in
the ingredients.

Steven X. Mills

**Awareness is creative
potential in an age where
distraction rules.**

To you, the user:

It is my sincere hope that you find wisdom, awareness and self-discovery throughout the pages of
this journal that will aid you on your continued
journey through life.

Introduction:

Keeping a journal of the foods we eat can help us to understand what our own diet is actually made up of, as opposed to our already formed pre-conceptions of what we 'think' we're putting into our bodies. This journal is designed to assist you in focusing on your own food mindfulness practice - the understanding of your own dietary habits and lifestyle. It is a visual tool to aid you in shifting from a re-active dietary stance to a pro-active, conscious super-consumer, by focusing not only on the foods you eat, but also the ingredients inside the products eaten.

What is Food Mindfulness?

Our daily lives are increasingly distractive and chaotic; the media which adorn the streets of our towns and cities, the devices in our pockets, our homes and our wrists, all collude to distract and interrupt our already over-loaded mind states with a cloud of constant confusion and mania. It is due in-part to this that, from early in the morning to late into the evening, our food choices are increasingly reactive, rushed and subconscious. They are often fuelled by an ever thirsting lust for high-fat high-sugar high-salt products, to hit that instant and forever-fleeting dopamine-fuelled sweet-spot within our tastebuds. These food items are easy to access and even easier to prepare, which undoubtably adds to our increased dependance on overly engineered, unnatural and manufactured dietary products as opposed to nutritionally dense whole foods.

It is through Food Mindfulness that we can counter-act this state of habitual dietary reactivity. By being mindful of the food, and the ingredients which make up our food, we can make our relationship with our diets measurable and therefore manageable. We can take pride in what we put into our body and re-assert gratitude into our food/body relationships. All it takes is a little dietary-orientated daily mindfulness training.

How do I use this journal for my Food Mindfulness practice?

It's simple. Record all food and beverages you consume through-out the duration of each day within the pages of this journal. Count and record next to each entry the amount of individual ingredients listed on the packet or packaging (if provided). At the end of each day, total up and make note of the amount of ingredients you have consumed, by adding together the ingredients from each individual entry.

You will find that typically, the more whole foods you consume, the fewer the sum of ingredients consumed will be.

The glasses of water icons on the right side of each page should also be used to record the amount of water you are consuming each day. Each symbol is designed to represent 500ml of water.

How many days should I do the journal for?

The journal is designed to last a month and consist of 31 journal entry pages. But it's completely up to you as an individual, how long you wish to continue keeping your food mindfulness journal. After you've completed this one, simply construct your own, or re-order another copy of the original journal.

Is this journal intended for weight-loss or weight-gain?

No. The goal of this food mindfulness journal is not to directly achieve variations in our body weight, but instead it is designed to be a tool to help us make conscious decisions in regards to the food we put into our bodies. However, when it's measurable, it's manageable, and once we're in control of our diets, we can manip-ulate them to achieve our wellness goals.

What do I do if I run out of space to record the things I have eaten?

If you run out of space, use the 'Notes' section at the back of the food journal to record any 'overflow' you may have. Just make sure to put the date at the start of the entry, so you don't get mixed up when referring back to it in future.

Food Mindfulness:
Ingredients

5	Root Vegetable Crisps
1	Banana
1	Porridge Oats
10	Oat Alternative to Milk
1	Apple
2	Crunchy Peanut Butter
1	Avocado
1	Organic Cinnamon Powder
1	Sweet Potato
1	Powdered Ginger
7	Apricot Jam
24	Seeded Batch Sliced Bread

Country: **United Kingdom**   Date: **19/02/19**

No. Ingredients Consumed: 55

No. Of Unknown Ingredients Consumed: 3

Water Level

Things To Consider Tomorrow: Drink more water.

Introduction:

What do I do with all the 'unknown' ingredients?

When you come across an unknown or mystery ingredient within your diet, you may want to explore its definition or origin. There's a specific section within this journal tailored for this purpose. Within the 'Ingredients Definitions' section, you will find space to explore, record and make notes of these items. Please see page 90 for an example of this.

Name: Pascale Davies

Start Date: 24/07/19

I am starting this journal because...

I would like to be more conscious with food & have a better understanding at whats going into my body PLUS impact on the environment.

Food Journal
And Diary

	2x Pitta bread
11	Vegan butter
5	Marmite
1	Lettice leaves
1	Spring onion
1	Celery
1	tomatoes
8	humus – all natural
15	Chutney – all natural
24	Vegan nuggets
	Sour snaks (whole pack)
	Bread
1	Oil
3	Vinigar
2	Olives – all natural
4	Potatoes w' rosmany, oil, salt ⟩ home cooked
5	Tomatoes, oil, salt, pepper, rosmary ⟩ cooked
6	Salad, all single ingredients, lettuce, celery, carrot, peas, yellow pepp
6	Dressing, oil, mustard, salt, pepper, sugar, vinig
1	Coffee
7	Oatmilk
1	Coffee

Country: _UK (ENGLAND)_   Date: _24/07/19_

7	Oatmilk
4	Milkshake, oatmilk & choc powder.
?	1x glass of rosé

No. Ingredients Consumed: _____

No. Of Unknown Ingredients Consumed: _Approx 21 - basically all the nuggets_

Bottles
Water Level   ▓ ▓ ▓ ▓ ▢ ▢ ▢ ▢

Things To Consider Tomorrow: _LESS SUGAR!_
Eat natural foods ☑

15

	2 x toast
11	Vegan butter
5	Marmite
8	Coffe w' oat milk

Country: ENGLAND　　　　　　　Date: 25/07/19

No. Ingredients Consumed: _____

No. Of Unknown Ingredients Consumed: _____

Water Level

Things To Consider Tomorrow: _____

Consumer Notes

Food Journal And Diary

Country: _____   Date: _____

No. Ingredients Consumed: _____

No. Of Unknown Ingredients Consumed: _____

Water Level   🥛 🥛 🥛 🥛 🥛 🥛 🥛 🥛

Things To Consider Tomorrow: _____

Consumer Notes

**Food Journal
And Diary**

Country: _____   Date: _____

No. Ingredients Consumed: _____

No. Of Unknown Ingredients Consumed: _____

Water Level   🥛 🥛 🥛 🥛 🥛 🥛 🥛 🥛

Things To Consider Tomorrow: _____

_____

Consumer Notes

**Food Journal
And Diary**

Country: _____   Date: _____

No. Ingredients Consumed: _____

No. Of Unknown Ingredients Consumed: _____

Water Level   ⬜ ⬜ ⬜ ⬜ ⬜ ⬜ ⬜ ⬜

Things To Consider Tomorrow: _____
_____

Consumer Notes

**Food Journal
And Diary**

Country: _____   Date: _____

No. Ingredients Consumed: _____

No. Of Unknown Ingredients Consumed: _____

Water Level   🥛 🥛 🥛 🥛 🥛 🥛 🥛 🥛

Things To Consider Tomorrow: _____

Consumer Notes

Food Journal And Diary

Country: _____   Date: _____

No. Ingredients Consumed: _____

No. Of Unknown Ingredients Consumed: _____

Water Level   🥛 🥛 🥛 🥛 🥛 🥛 🥛 🥛

Things To Consider Tomorrow: _____
_____

Food Journal
And Diary

Country: _____   Date: _____

No. Ingredients Consumed: _____

No. Of Unknown Ingredients Consumed: _____

Water Level   🥛 🥛 🥛 🥛 🥛 🥛 🥛 🥛

Things To Consider Tomorrow: _____

_____

Consumer Notes

**Food Journal
And Diary**

Country: _____   **Date:** _____

No. Ingredients Consumed: _____

No. Of Unknown Ingredients Consumed: _____

Water Level   ▽ ▽ ▽ ▽ ▽ ▽ ▽ ▽

Things To Consider Tomorrow: _____

Consumer Notes

Food Journal And Diary

Country: _____   Date: _____

No. Ingredients Consumed: _____

No. Of Unknown Ingredients Consumed: _____

Water Level   ⬚ ⬚ ⬚ ⬚ ⬚ ⬚ ⬚ ⬚

Things To Consider Tomorrow: _____

Consumer Notes

**Food Journal
And Diary**

Country: _____   Date: _____

No. Ingredients Consumed: _____

No. Of Unknown Ingredients Consumed: _____

Water Level   ▯ ▯ ▯ ▯ ▯ ▯ ▯ ▯

Things To Consider Tomorrow: _____

Consumer Notes

**Food Journal
And Diary**

Country: _____   Date: _____

No. Ingredients Consumed: _____

No. Of Unknown Ingredients Consumed: _____

Water Level ⬜ ⬜ ⬜ ⬜ ⬜ ⬜ ⬜ ⬜

Things To Consider Tomorrow: _____

Consumer Notes

**Food Journal
And Diary**

Country: _____   Date: _____

No. Ingredients Consumed: _____

No. Of Unknown Ingredients Consumed: _____

Water Level   ⊔ ⊔ ⊔ ⊔ ⊔ ⊔ ⊔ ⊔

Things To Consider Tomorrow: _____

Consumer Notes

Food Journal And Diary

Country: _____   Date: _____

No. Ingredients Consumed: _____

No. Of Unknown Ingredients Consumed: _____

Water Level   ▯ ▯ ▯ ▯ ▯ ▯ ▯ ▯

Things To Consider Tomorrow: _____

Consumer Notes

Food Journal And Diary

Country: _____   Date: _____

No. Ingredients Consumed: _____

No. Of Unknown Ingredients Consumed: _____

Water Level   ▢ ▢ ▢ ▢ ▢ ▢ ▢ ▢

Things To Consider Tomorrow: _____

Consumer Notes

Food Journal And Diary

Country: _____   Date: _____

No. Ingredients Consumed: _____

No. Of Unknown Ingredients Consumed: _____

Water Level   🥛 🥛 🥛 🥛 🥛 🥛 🥛 🥛

Things To Consider Tomorrow: _____
_____

Consumer Notes

**Food Journal
And Diary**

Country: _____   Date: _____

No. Ingredients Consumed: _____

No. Of Unknown Ingredients Consumed: _____

Water Level   🥛 🥛 🥛 🥛 🥛 🥛 🥛 🥛

Things To Consider Tomorrow: _____

Food Journal
And Diary

Country: _____   **Date:** _____

No. Ingredients Consumed: _____

No. Of Unknown Ingredients Consumed: _____

Water Level ⬜ ⬜ ⬜ ⬜ ⬜ ⬜ ⬜ ⬜

Things To Consider Tomorrow: _____

_____

Consumer Notes

**Food Journal
And Diary**

Country: _____   Date: _____

No. Ingredients Consumed: _____

No. Of Unknown Ingredients Consumed: _____

Water Level   🥛 🥛 🥛 🥛 🥛 🥛 🥛 🥛

Things To Consider Tomorrow: _____

Consumer Notes

**Food Journal
And Diary**

Country: _____ Date: _____

No. Ingredients Consumed: _____

No. Of Unknown Ingredients Consumed: _____

Water Level   ▯ ▯ ▯ ▯ ▯ ▯ ▯ ▯

Things To Consider Tomorrow: _____

_____

Consumer Notes

Food Journal
And Diary

Country: _____   Date: _____

No. Ingredients Consumed: _____

No. Of Unknown Ingredients Consumed: _____

Water Level   🥛 🥛 🥛 🥛 🥛 🥛 🥛 🥛

Things To Consider Tomorrow: _____
_____

Consumer Notes

**Food Journal
And Diary**

Country: _____   Date: _____

No. Ingredients Consumed: ....

No. Of Unknown Ingredients Consumed: ....

Water Level   ⊔ ⊔ ⊔ ⊔ ⊔ ⊔ ⊔ ⊔

Things To Consider Tomorrow: _____

_____

Consumer Notes

Food Journal And Diary

Country: _____   Date: _____

No. Ingredients Consumed: _____

No. Of Unknown Ingredients Consumed: _____

Water Level   🥛 🥛 🥛 🥛 🥛 🥛 🥛 🥛

Things To Consider Tomorrow: _____

Consumer Notes

Food Journal
And Diary

Country: _____   Date: _____

No. Ingredients Consumed: _____

No. Of Unknown Ingredients Consumed: _____

Water Level   ⊔ ⊔ ⊔ ⊔ ⊔ ⊔ ⊔ ⊔

Things To Consider Tomorrow: _____

Consumer Notes

Food Journal
And Diary

Country: _____   **Date:** _____

No. Ingredients Consumed: _____

No. Of Unknown Ingredients Consumed: _____

Water Level   ⬜ ⬜ ⬜ ⬜ ⬜ ⬜ ⬜ ⬜

Things To Consider Tomorrow: _____

_____

Consumer Notes

**Food Journal
And Diary**

Country: _____   **Date:** _____

No. Ingredients Consumed: _____

No. Of Unknown Ingredients Consumed: _____

Water Level   ⊔ ⊔ ⊔ ⊔ ⊔ ⊔ ⊔ ⊔

Things To Consider Tomorrow: _____

_____

Consumer Notes

Food Journal
And Diary

Country: _____   Date: _____

No. Ingredients Consumed: _____

No. Of Unknown Ingredients Consumed: _____

Water Level   ⊔ ⊔ ⊔ ⊔ ⊔ ⊔ ⊔ ⊔

Things To Consider Tomorrow: _____

_____

Consumer Notes

Food Journal
And Diary

Country: _____   Date: _____

No. Ingredients Consumed: _____

No. Of Unknown Ingredients Consumed: _____

Water Level   🥛 🥛 🥛 🥛 🥛 🥛 🥛 🥛

Things To Consider Tomorrow: _____

_____

Consumer Notes

**Food Journal
And Diary**

Country: _____   Date: _____

No. Ingredients Consumed: _____

No. Of Unknown Ingredients Consumed: _____

Water Level   ⬜ ⬜ ⬜ ⬜ ⬜ ⬜ ⬜ ⬜

Things To Consider Tomorrow: _____

Consumer Notes

Food Journal
And Diary

Country: _____   Date: _____

No. Ingredients Consumed: _____

No. Of Unknown Ingredients Consumed: _____

Water Level   🥛 🥛 🥛 🥛 🥛 🥛 🥛 🥛

Things To Consider Tomorrow: _____
_____

Consumer Notes

Food Journal And Diary

Country: _____   **Date:** _____

No. Ingredients Consumed: _____

No. Of Unknown Ingredients Consumed: _____

Water Level   ⬜ ⬜ ⬜ ⬜ ⬜ ⬜ ⬜ ⬜

Things To Consider Tomorrow: _____

_____

Additional Notes

Date: _____

Additional Notes:

Date:

Additional Notes:

Date: _____

Additional Notes:

Additional Notes:

Additional Notes:

Date: _____

Additional Notes:

Additional Notes:

Date: _____

Additional Notes:

Date: _____

Additional Notes:

Date: _____

Additional Notes:

Ingredient Definitions

Name of Item	Definition/Description	Found Within
E472e	Mono- and diacetyltartaric acid esters of mono- and diglycerides of fatty acids	Seeded Batch Sliced Bread
	Esters of synthetic fats, produced from natural fatty acids found within animals and plants. E472e is mostly sourced from plants, however not always. The product is commonly mixed with other components and has a composition similar to partially digested natural fats.	
	Most commonly used for strengthening dough by building a stronger glutenous bond.	

Ingredients Definitions

Name of Item	Definition/Description	Found Within

Ingredients Definitions

Name of Item	Definition/Description	Found Within

Ingredients Definitions

!

Name of Item	Definition/Description	Found Within

Ingredients Definitions

Name of Item	Definition/Description	Found Within

Ingredients Definitions

Name of Item	Definition/Description	Found Within

Ingredients Definitions

Name of Item	Definition/Description	Found Within

Ingredients Definitions

Name of Item	Definition/Description	Found Within

Ingredients Definitions

!

Name of Item	Definition/Description	Found Within

Ingredients Definitions

!

Name of Item	Definition/Description	Found Within

Ingredients Definitions

Name of Item	Definition/Description	Found Within

Ingredients Definitions

!

Name of Item	Definition/Description	Found Within

Congratulations

First of all, congratulations on becoming one of the elite few who has taken ownership of their food consumption. And a massive thank you for choosing this journal as a resource to help you on your journey of dietary awareness and understanding. I hope that you will finish this document having expanded your knowledge of your own diet, and have learned something new, beneficial and awakening.

If you wish to continue this food mindfulness practice, I encourage you to undertake the construction and implementation of your own structures and approaches to food-mindfulness. Through developing personalised charts and forms, you will find yourself more emotionally invested in the practice and may find it easier to continue on your mindful eating pathway. If you wish to simply re-peat this exercise, to discover some things you might have missed or simply to monitor how this practice might change over time, the purchase of a second copy would be greatly appreciated.

I wish you all the best in your on-going and future life practices, and hope that being mindful of the ingredients you consume will change your view of the world the way it has changed mine.

End Notes

Disclaimer:

By purchasing or using this journal or products and services related to Consumer Notes: Food Journal and Diary you are voluntarily accepting all parts of this disclaimer.

Not a Doctor:

This journal makes no health or medical claims regarding the interpretation or use of any information contained or recorded by the user within this journal.

The information and structure provided within this journal and related products and services are for self-discovery and informal purposes only, and are made available to the reader as a self-help tool. Therefore the author takes no responsibility for any actions or consequences which may occur as a result of using this journal or any related content.

The structure provided within this journal is strictly experimental. It is only intended as a tool for the user to explore their familiarity and relationship with the ingredients contained within the food they choose to consume.

For medical, psychological and nutritional advice please seek the advice of a qualified professional. The author has no trained medical, psychological or nutritional background, and does not claim to do so.

If you feel you are developing or suffering from a diet-related condition/eating disorder, please seek professional medical advice immediately.

You are Responsible:

The user/reader is responsible for all personal choices or actions made before, during or after the use of the Food Journal and Diary or any related content both online and offline. The user/reader should be aware that they are liable as a whole for their own actions, and the author/publisher will not accept liability in the rare case that any form of illness or death occur as a result of using this product and/or related services.

The user/reader acknowledges that they take full responsibility for their own health, life and wellbeing, including all decisions made in the present and in the future.

No Guarantees:

The goal of the author is primarily, if nothing else, to assist you in increasing your awareness of the ingredients contained within your diet, and build awareness. The author does not intend this journal to be used for weight loss. You may experience a feeling that you want to cut down the amount of ingredients in your diet, by consuming more whole foods, as a side-effect of using this journal. This is not guaranteed by the author and the author will take no liability for this potential outcome. The success of this journal, whatever your reason for using it, will depend greatly on your own effort, motivation, commitment and follow-through. These are all things you (the user/reader) should accept all responsibility for.

Borrowing:

Eating Disorders and Food
Mindfulness:

Whilst food mindfulness and awareness can be a life changing tool
to put into your tool chest, it would be damaging, ignorant and ne-
glectful to not acknowledge the various common eating disorders
which can develop in-part from an over-examination of diet.

Eating disorders are mental conditions which can effect people of
all age, race and body types, and can lead to significant ill health
with long lasting Effects, even after a recover has been made from
the initial disorder.

The three most common eating disorders noted by the UK's National Health Service, as stated in the Guidelines for GPs and Other
Professionals: Eating Disorders, are anorexia nervosa, bulimia nervosa and binge eating disorder, however there are many others.

It is worth while to take the time to familiarise yourself with these
three disorders, so that you can identify, recognise and understand
the symptoms should you need to in the future.

Eating Disorders:

Anorexia nervosa is categorised by an individual maintaining a
body weight of less than 15% below the expected for their par-
ticular hight, combined with an extreme 'fear of fatness', distorted
body image influenced by weight and shape, and self-induced
weight loss methods. This may be a voluntary avoidance to food,
self-induced vomiting, purging, excessive exercise or use of appetite suppressants.

A person suffering from bulimia nervosa may undergo repeat episodes of overeating of large quantities of food, where the individual feels as if they cannot stop eating or have control of how much
they are consuming. This is often combined with compensatory
periods of behaviours to prevent weight gain such as self-induced

vomiting, appetite suppressants, fasting, laxatives and other diet effecting drugs. The individual will also suffer from fluctuations in self-esteem influenced by their body weight and/or shape.

Binge eating disorder is the newest of the three most recognised conditions. It is categorised by individuals who have episodes of overeating large amounts of food, where the person feels out of control in relation to their food consumption both in quantity and food choice. These 'binge' eating episodes usually continue until the individual feels uncomfortably full. Other symptoms of binge eating disorder also include eating large quantities of food when they are not even hungry, eating noticeably faster than the considered norm, eating alone due to embarrassment or fear of judgment, and feeling disgusted, depressed or guilty after a binge period.

Help:

If you are concerned that you, a close friend or loved one are suffering or struggling with an eating disorder please seek out adequate professional medical advice. It is noted within the UK's National Health Service's Guidelines for GPs and Other Professionals: Eating Disorders, that early diagnosis and intervention is directly related to improved outcomes for in patients.

It is also worth noting that some sufferers of these conditions may actively avoid detection and therefore help. So the actual diagnosis of eating disorders can sometimes prove challenging and problematic.

Feedback:

For inquires, to start a conversation or to provide feedback, please contact:

consumernotesservices@gmail.com

We'd love to hear from you!

Please note:

Emails are checked and responded to once weekly on Mondays. This is so we can use our time and energy more effectively, in order to produce the best possible products and resources to serve our customers better. Thank you in advance for being patient and understanding.

You can also give us a review on Amazon.

Thank you for choosing this Food Journal and Diary.

Printed in Great Britain
by Amazon